TABLE OF CONTENTS

FOREWORD
Why Read This Boring Little Book?

Greetings! My name is Dr Thomas Bowen and I am an Orthodontist. I love what I do and we have made it our core focus to help everyone, "REACH THEIR SMILE" You may be wondering why you should take the time to read this little book. I wrote this book to help answer some questions and provide some clarity about what Orthodontics is about and why it is so important. Besides, this book is really short and easy to read. You opened this book to learn about orthodontic treatment an how to make a good decision for yourself or your family.

Just a short bit of information about the author of this book...ME. Most orthodontists attend four years of dental school and then go directly into their residency training of 2-3 years to become an orthodontist. My journey to become an orthodontist was a little, let's say unconventional. I attended four years of dental school after college to become a dentist. Instead of becoming an orthodontist after that I practiced as a general dentist. First as a captain in the USArmy Dental Corps and then in my own private practice for ten years. During that time in private practice, one of my mentors who I worked with in the Army left his private practice to become an orthodontist. His move had a lot of influence on me to explore the possibility of pursuing orthodontics. And that's what I did. I sold my practice and spend 2 and a half years training to specialize and become an orthodontist. So I bring a pretty strong background of years of performing general dentistry as well as my specialty as an orthodontist

Enough about me. This book is about you, the parent and your son or daughter. It will provide information you need to know to make intelligent, responsible decisions about your child's health, appearance, self-esteem and social interactions...of a permanent lifelong nature. There is an abundance of information (and mis-information) about braces and orthodontics out there. Even so, many families are still a little confused when it comes to knowing when they should see an orthodontist, how to choose the best orthodontic provider for their family and understanding how the orthodontic process works. There are some major misconceptions out there about braces that I thought I would address right now.

To start, we are no longer dealing with heavy, ugly tight and painful metal braces to move the teeth. The experience won't be anything like it was

REACH YOUR
SMILE

A Guide to Orthodontics for Children and Adults

QUIZ:
What is Most Important to You in Selecting an Orthodontist?

Dr. Thomas B. Bowen, DMD

Reach Your Smile: A Guide to Orthodontics
for Children and Adults

ISBN: 978-1-970095-14-2

when you were a kid. Braces are smaller, more comfortable placed on the teeth very easily. The wires today are much more comfortable, more effective and efficient. The days painful adjustments, frequent visits, and long appointments are over. Todays orthodontic technology is comfortable, often allows for extended office visit intervals and provides for quick appointments that easily fit into your day.

Secondly, the aesthetics have dramatically changed for the better. Gone is the stigma of being called "metal mouth" and 'train tracks" Modern appliances for orthodontics blend nicely into the teeth(including the invisible ones) Orthodontics is well accepted as a normal part of growing up. Most kids will think it is COOL to have braces. Now for those kids and adults who do not want metal, we can move teeth without any brackets or wires, almost invisibly. We can use clear aligners to straighten teeth. You are probably aware of invisible braces, maybe have heard of the brand, Invisalign. They are one of many companies that fabricate clear aligners that are worn to move teeth. Now we can achieve more certain results and sometimes in a shorter period of time than with braces.

Third, orthodontic treatment has also become more affordable than ever. With many offices offering extended financing options, accepting flexible spending account payments and customizing payment plans to make orthodontics fit into their budget. The rigid payment structures and high down payments are a thing of the past. Today, finances should not be a barrier in preventing anyone from REACHING THEIR SMILE.

I believe an orthodontic journey for a family should be about more than just teeth, which is easily forgotten in todays hectic, aesthetic-forward society. Orthodontics is about creating a healthy, functional bite to last the rest of your life. Straight teeth function better, are easier to clean and are more likely to last a lifetime. People with straight teeth can avoid gum disease, which can have serious health ramifications.

Properly aligned jaws may reduce the risk of temporomandibular joint disorders(TMJ) which can ruin sleep or cause chronic headaches of migraines. Both kids and adults with great smiles feel better about themselves and that can greatly increase their confidence. It's also about teamwork, forming trust, and fostering mutual respect among your family, your orthodontist, and the office team. It's about realizing there's a living, breathing unique human attached to those pearly whites. Its about giving your child's confidence room to grow and letting their personality shine!

I've listed below the 10 most common questions that families ask us during their initial visit. The chapters of this book are laid out to address these questions.

1. Why should I even see an orthodontist

2. When should my child see an orthodontist

3. Why can't we just see my dentist? Why an orthodontist?

4. How do I chose between orthodontist?

5. What can I expect at the Initial Consultation and exam?

6. Will my child need teeth removed?

7. What will the braces experience be like?

8. What are the treatment options that are available other than braces?

9. How can I make orthodontic care fit into my family budget?

10. What happens when the braces come off?

If you already know the answers to these questions, you can put this book down. Either you're an orthodontist already or have super mental psychic powers!
If you don't know the answers to them and/or hesitant to visit the orthodontist, then this book is exactly what you need to help. Like I said, this is a relatively short easy to read book that has minimal technical/medical jargon.

Throughout this book, we will go into a little more detail answering each of the above questions, as well as give you some bonus material at the end. When you're finished, you'll have enough solid information to embark on your child's smile journey as a well-informed, confident parent.

Dr. Thomas Bowen, DMD

CHAPTER 1

Why is My Child's Smile So Important?

If you are weighing the yes/no and now/later decisions of orthodontic care or braces, you'll be trying to decide just how important or unimportant it really is.

Some parents feel "looks aren't everything." Some think their kid should just be tough-minded about this and not overly sensitive. Some may not have had orthodontic care when they were children and think, *Hey, I turned out just fine. I have a great spouse, a good career, friends—so what's the big deal?*

But that was then. This is *now:* the age of social media.

Social shaming and bullying is a lot worse, a lot more common, and a lot more persistent than when you were a kid. Teen suicide is on the rise, and such suicides share one thing in common: shocked and bewildered parents who could not conceive of their child ending his own life. Sure, they might've noticed he was a *little* depressed. They knew he was being bullied and spending more time home, alone, not leaving his room, but geez, he *is* a teenager, after all. What once was a few days or weeks of misery contained in the cafeteria with a few bullies is now endless, expansive, and broadcast online to everybody. Behind a computer screen, it can get far nastier than most would dare in person. Sometimes, kids bully each other for no reason, being a buck-toothed girl or a boy with gaps in between their teeth is enough to exacerbate the situation.

Signs Your Child May Be Being Bullied

- Decrease in self-esteem
- Not wanting to go to school
- Skipping school
- Injuries they can't explain
- Self-destructive behaviors
  (e.g., harming themselves)
- Declining school grades
- Sleep difficulties
- Loss of interest in schoolwork or activities
- Sudden loss of friends or avoiding social groups
- Changes in eating habits

A straight, clean and healthy smile can not only give your child the confidence she needs to embrace her true worth but can also pave the way toward easier socialization at school, church, or during extracurricular activities. Do your child a favor and talk about her smile and how it might be affecting her.

Beyond that, there's a life ahead of your child. Going to junior high with crooked teeth and a humiliating smile is one thing. Hey, plenty of kids are going to school *without shoes* for heaven's sake. But going to college admission interviews, packing up and heading off to college, going to job interviews, trying to fit into new and anxiety-rich environments at a faraway college or new workplace with a bad smile—and maybe unavoidable bad breath with it—and daytime headaches from nighttime teeth-grinding is a lot more serious.

This isn't *just* a cosmetic issue. Misaligned, crooked teeth equal *significant* medical problems.

Poorly aligned teeth can produce chronic headaches and migraines, contribute to digestive problems because of the inability to properly chew foods, and make getting a decent night's sleep impossible. Maybe most dangerous of all, it can foster gum disease. Gum disease has absolute links to diabetes, heart disease, strokes and dementia, as well as, of course, the loss of natural teeth altogether. Orthodontic corrections later in adult life are more difficult; they can be painful, require time off work, and at best, they'll just be embarrassing. *Invisible braces aren't really totally invisible, and you're thirty-eight? Forty-four? Fifty-one? C'mon.*

Uncorrected mouth problems and misaligned teeth make for strangely stretched gums inevitably destined to separate from teeth. This could allow "pockets" for infections and periodontal disease to arise and turn into very difficult, painful, and costly problems late in life.

In the teenage years, failure to spend even $4,000 can easily create a $40,000 full mouth restoration case at age forty or fifty or embarrassing, health-compromising removal of all teeth and use of dentures at age sixty.

Gum disease is serious business. It worsens the risks of and heightens dangers from diabetes, heart disease, strokes, and dementia. Ignoring preteen or teen teeth misalignment may virtually guarantee adult medical problems. If there is a genetic history of any of these medical problems I just named, you only worsen the odds of your son or daughter suffering from them by ignoring or postponing needed orthodontic treatment.

Aside from impacting health, a poorly aligned smile can significantly impact your child's comfort. Headaches, toothaches, sinus problems, dry mouth, snoring, drooling, bad breath, and insomnia are all symptoms of a smile that isn't straight, jaws that aren't aligned, or teeth that are too close together or not quite close enough. Oftentimes, however, the mouth is the last place we check for signs of discomfort, loss of sleep, or even a simple headache.

If your child's pediatrician can't figure out why she's not sleeping well or experiencing headaches or even insomnia for which there seems to be no cause, a simple thirty-minute exam at your local orthodontist could provide a clear solution in no time!

Here is what I'm told by an awful lot of parents:

> *"I had wonderful parents, but I sure wish they had found a way to afford the braces I needed and gotten me the care I needed when I was a kid, so I didn't grow up to have this bad smile my whole life."*

And what I hear from almost every adult patient getting orthodontic treatment and braces is:

> *"I had wonderful parents, but I sure wish they had found a way to afford the braces I needed and gotten me the care I needed when I was a kid, so I didn't grow up to have this bad smile my whole life and have all these problems now."*

Is this how you want your daughter or son talking about you ten, twenty, or thirty years from now? Is this how you want them remembering their childhood? Your parenting?

If that sounds pretty damned pushy, I admit: it is. I kept it in the book for the very simple reason that this is *truly* what I have heard so much over the years, and I am sincere about letting you reflect on it. All parents want to do the right thing. They don't want to let their children down in any way, and I'm sure you don't either.

You know, parents just about kill themselves over their kids' college, trying their best to guide the decision, trekking around the country on campus visits, worrying over campus culture, or taking on *serious* debt. Every parent understands what many kids can't—that it's not about the few years of college but rather the forty or fifty years afterward.

I assure you, this is the same. It's not about the bad, humiliating smile and bad bite transformed now, for high school. It's about the many, many years to come. They really can't appreciate that now, but *you* can.

No parent wants their child to suffer, either from teeth that actually hurt, headaches you can't explain, insomnia that affects their daily life, or insecurity your child may be feeling because of a crooked or oversized smile.

The fact is, your child's formative years are actually the most sensitive for his or her teeth. Now is the time to pay close attention to your child's smile, behavior, peer relationships, and confidence level.

If any or all are lacking, a qualified orthodontist may help give you and your child the peace of mind you both crave.

The Top 5 Reasons People Avoid Seeing the Orthodontist

1. Patients are afraid it's going to hurt.
Pain is the number-one reason most people avoid going to the orthodontist. However, modern technology—and choosing the right orthodontist—can ensure that your child enjoys a pain-free orthodontic experience.

2. Patients are afraid it's going to cost too much. Not only are most orthodontic procedures more affordable than ever, but insurance, payment plans and a variety of other financing options make this all but a moot point for most of my patients. Remember, orthodontists aren't in this to get rich, they're here to make sure your child's teeth, smile, and jaw are aligned to make his or her life better—period! We're not going to let something like price get in the way of creating a better, safer, healthier smile for your child.

3. Patients are afraid it's going to take too long / miss too much school or work. Regardless of the type of orthodontic procedure your child needs, time is of the essence. Modern technology and ease of access allows us to work around your child's school schedule with minimal absences. After initial visits, and barring the actual procedure itself, most visits and/or adjustments are routine and can take anywhere from fifteen to forty-five minutes.

4. Patients do not see the need to take action. Eroding, crooked or unaligned smiles can take time to happen, but the time to act is now. Orthodontic irregularities don't just heal on their own or disappear if you ignore them. Your child's smile and overall dental health are too important to ignore out of questions of pain, convenience, or even price.

5. Patients have been treated in the past with an attitude of indifference. Let's face it, not all doctors are created equal. Every profession has its "bad apples," and to say dentistry is the exception would be to write fiction instead of fact. There is no room for indifference when it comes to your child's healthcare. Find an orthodontic specialist that offers not only state of the art technology for your child but state of the art service as well. Orthodontic specialists know what it's like to sit in the chair, and should provide every opportunity for patients, especially our younger patients, to feel comfortable, safe, and secure in our care.

Call us at 573-212-8723 or go to www.bowenortho.com to schedule your own Customized Smile Analysis.

CHAPTER 2

When Should My Child See an Orthodontist?

Anterior Crossbite

Posterior Crossbite

Crowding

Open Bite
An open bite is usually due to an oral habit

Protrusion

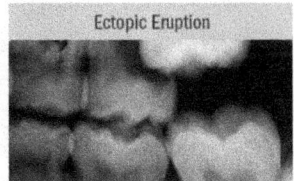
Ectopic Eruption
Ectopically erupting maxillary molar

Complete Class III

Diastema

Oral Habits

Take a look at the pictures above. These are all issues that represent non-ideal bites. Left untreated, they have potential to lead to issues with tooth development, jaw alignment, gum issues, or social concerns. Not all of these problems need orthodontic care immediately, but they are should be evaluated by an orthodontist sooner rather than later.

The American Association of Orthodontists recommends that kids have their first orthodontic check-up by a licensed orthodontist starting at age 7 or 8. Orthodontists are just looking out for the best interest of your child to avoid serious dental problems and, when indicated keep treatment easy, painless, more predictable.

Now there may be some over-prescribing and premature prescribing by some doctors. There are bad apples in every orchard. We only recommend early treatment to a small percentage of patients that exhibit some of the problems as shown in the previous picture. There is a very legitimate, clinically documented and 90 percent of the time, clearly visible reason why some kids need orthodontic treatment and care at this age: malocclusion.

Malocclusion is mostly genetic, so if your son or daughter has it, blame their grandparents. It's a fancy-pants term for all things related to misaligned teeth. Teeth growing angled, crooked, and into a too crowded space. It can be a single tooth, a few teeth, or the whole mouth. There can be causes too, like early premature loss of primary teeth, chronic thumb-sucking, or even an accident the seemed to leave no lasting effect at its moment in time.

Here are a few examples of things that should be evaluated by and orthodontic specialist sooner rather than later.

- Crossbites: A crossbite occurs when the jaw deviated to one side with an improper fit of the upper and lower teeth from left to right or front to back. Crossbites cam lead to worn and chipped teeth, jaw pain and asymmetric growth of the jaws. Left untreated, the crossbite will require more extensive treatment later in life and significant jaw surgery in most cases.

- Thumb-sucking: thumb-sucking habits beginning at the age of seven or older should be corrected immediately in order to prevent severe jaw alignment problems.

- Permanent teeth that are growing into the wrong spots

- Severely protruded front teeth at risk for injury or causing teasing at school, and:

- Severe crowding with permanent teeth erupting into poor quality gum tissue.

With any of these situations, we can discuss the pros and cons of early intervention and treatment versus waiting until all the permanent teeth are in for braces. If you are anxious about the appearance of you child's teeth or your child is self-conscious about his or her appearance, early treatment might be the best choice. Not only are most orthodontic problems more difficult to correct later, but self-image and personality inhibition can be hard for a person to leave behind.

Having malocclusion does not guarantee a child will need braces. That is one of the thing that worries me about nonspecialists like family dentist substituting themselves for orthodontist, and parents letting it happen. They easily miss an early diagnosis of malocclusion when it could have been averted without braces. Or they may leap to braces as the only way to treat all malocclusion.

Not having that first orthodontic exam at 7 or 8(no later than 9) will have serious consequences, often requiring more treatment and higher costs later in life. What most parents fail to realize is these treatment problems for many kids are urgent and should be treated as such.

If your child does need braces-now or at some predictable future time-the outcome of the exam can lead to sensible decisions. If not now, treatment to prevent the need can begin, and also, you can begin saving money for braces or other procedures if necessary later on in you child's life. It may give you time to save. Utilizing a Health Savings Account or Flex Spending Account can help as well.

Let me be clear. I am not in the business of putting braces on any child who doesn't need braces. My office is not a braces store. I'm in the business of helping kids and families get this right. I want them to get the right treatment, when and if they are ready. I want them to have as perfect a smile and as few oral health problems as possible. I make sure my patients are informed- that's why I wrote this information and put together this book.

Kids do need braces, but not all kids and certainly not the same braces for all. Some kids are better served by other orthodontic treatments instead of or before bracers. We will collaborate, you and I, to figure out what is or isn't needed and what options are best if there is a need for your child.

CHAPTER 3

Sleep Disordered Breathing (SDB) Problems

I wanted to talk about something that you may not think falls under the scope of orthodontic treatment. These fall under the the topic of sleep breathing disorders. This chapter will give some general causes, symptoms and seeing another benefit to seeing the orthodontist at an early age can benefit

Chronic snoring and chronic mouth-breathing in kids is not normal, and may indicate a small airway and a higher potential for sleep apnea as an adult. Research is clear that kids with breathing issues and not getting enough oxygen during sleep hours are prone to a host of negative associations with their body and brain development, including bed-wetting, sleep-walking, diminished growth, hormonal, metabolic problems. 25% of ADHD problems are children deprived of restful sleep, thus behavior problems.

As parents, you can do a couple really quick things to help assess if your child may have a suspected breathing issue during sleep. First, ask yourself the following six questions

1. Does my child snore frequently?

2. Does my child usually sleep through the night, awake sleepy, or tire easily?

3. Does my child sound "nasally" when speaking?

4. Does my child have problems focusing in school?

5. Does my child grind his/her teeth?

6. Does my child get frequent headaches?

7. Does my child wet the bed?

Secondly, take a look in you child mouth and have them say' AHHHH" Look at the size of their tonsils and see if they look enlarged to you filling up the back of the throat.

Orthodontists, if they see the children early enough(such as 7-8, or earlier) can appropriately evaluate and suggest an approach, if indicated to help get children breathing better and minimize any detrimental impacts on their growth and life. Children my benefit from a home sleep study, or see an otolaryngologist(ENT) if large tonsils or adenoids need to be removed. Some simply need allery meds. A common approach may be simple upper jaw orthopedic expansion to correct narrow jaw, or lower jaw lengthening with widening of the dental arches. Within weeks/months the child typically rest better and awakens normally.

This chapter is not meant to scare you as parents, as many kids truly do not have any breathing issues, especially not those related to orthodontics. However, since an orthodontist can easily let you know if there is an issue with a quick check-up, and there usually not a charge to do so, it doesn't hurt to be proactive and get your child evaluated-especially if you are noticing an issue.

CHAPTER 4

Why Not Just a Dentist? Why an Orthodontist?

You undoubtedly already have a dentist.

Gee, isn't seeing an orthodontist going to cost a lot more?

I'm busy. More appointments?

Do I really need to get orthodontic check-ups for my kids?

Don't worry, these are all reasonable questions! It is true that, today, quite a few dentists dance over into our territory, and although they're not permitted to claim they're the same as orthodontists or provide orthodontic treatment (beware any who do), they're able to do things like provide Invisalign and other braces. This can be confusing. Here are the facts.

All orthodontists are dentists and we all graduate from the same dental schools. True enough. But that's where it stops for dentists. Orthodontists go to school for an additional two to three years to become credentialed specialists at diagnosing and providing the best treatment for conditions like:

- Difficulties chewing or biting
- Constant biting into the cheek, gums, or roof of the mouth
- Teeth that meet abnormally or don't meet at all
- Teeth grinding or clenching
- Crowded, misplaced or blocked out teeth
- Early or late loss of teeth
- Teeth grown in badly
- Teeth that protrude
- Embarrassing personal appearance due to teeth
- Facial imbalances
- Teeth or jaw misalignment, TMJ
- Chronic headaches and migraine
- Poor sleep
- Speech difficulties (that may never be outgrown or may develop later)

These are not dental care issues. They are orthodontic issues.

For *some* things, a generalist or jack-of-all-trades will do. For other things, you know it's smart to seek out the best specialist you can afford.

For example, if all your income is in a single W-2 from one employer and you have simple, ordinary deductions, getting your taxes prepared for the cheapest fee at the seasonal H&R Block office that opens up in your neighborhood shopping center is probably fine. But if you have W-2, 1099 and investment income from real estate, depreciation on real estate in several states, own stocks and you raise iguanas as a money hobby, you're going to get yourself a really good accountant, probably a CPA.

If you need the simplest will, leaving everything first to spouse or second to daughter may be okay. But if you are of some means and have several children and maybe also grandchildren as well as charities, you're going to need to see an *estate planning attorney*: not just any attorney—they all went to the same law schools—but a *specialist in estate planning*.

This is no different.

There are a few things to keep in mind when differentiating between a general dentist and an orthodontic specialist.

First, generalists or jacks-of-all-trades tend to work with one-size-fits-all, off-the-rack, standardized solutions. They may be limited to doing only what the computer dictates that they do, without bringing expertise and expert judgment to bear. They're often working with products from only one provider, without being able to select from a full range of options that would work best for you. Specialists, instead, tend to individually and carefully diagnose needs and provide personalized solutions.

Second, generalists and their use of inexpertly applied, standardized solutions tend to be cheaper than the fees of a specialist, but that also places economic pressure on them to do the treatment as quickly and simply as possible, because they've "cut it thin."

In this case, it's worth remembering that the treatment provided has permanent, lifelong, and life-impacting consequences. This concerns your health, future dental or jaw alignment or misalignment issues affecting quality of sleep (which can affect weight, even onset and management of type 2 diabetes and heart disease), as well as self-esteem and social and career success.

General Dentist. A general dentist gives routine checkups, preventative measures, cleans teeth, and fixes cavities. They may not start seeing children until they are seven to ten years old.

Pediatric Dentist. A pediatric dentist has two to three years of specialized education beyond dental school. They specialize in providing dental care to children and adolescents, offering checkups, preventative measures, cleanings, and cavities.

Orthodontist. An orthodontist has two to three years of specialized education beyond dental school and is an expert at straightening teeth and aligning the jaws. They assess patients and determine the best treatment route to straighten their teeth and align their jaws.

If you can, you want to choose an orthodontist for orthodontic care.

You may ask, *how do I know my doctor is an orthodontist?* It's a good question and a critical one to ask as you seek additional treatment for your child's dental issues.

Only orthodontists can belong to the American Association of Orthodontists (AAO). If you're looking for a local orthodontist, go online and visit **www.braces.org** to find a specialist in your area. This website features not only a searchable database of orthodontists but educational tips, answers and resources to help you on your quest for your child's healthiest smile!

Alternatively, you can ask your doctor if he or she has completed a two-to three-year residency in orthodontics and check with your state dental board to follow up on his reply. Dentists and orthodontists in most states will be registered differently with the dental board.

Do your homework; be a "dental detective" while on the hunt for such vital information. Look for the words "dental specialist in orthodontics" or ask your general dentist for a referral to a specialist. In urban and suburban areas, it will take minimal effort to find a specialist. In more remote, rural locations, your search might take you to another city or town. Don't be afraid to ask your dentist if an orthodontist travels to your town every month to see patients. There's a chance an orthodontist from a larger city comes to your town and works out of another dental office once or twice per month. Looking around can save valuable driving time and money.

One note: there is no disrespect between orthodontists and dentists. As a matter of fact, many orthodontic patients are referred by their dentists. These are great, capable, and caring professionals who know where their expertise begins and ends, and do not let ego or income opportunity step in front of what they know is best for their patients. Just as the family doctor refers his patients with possible or significant heart disease issues to a cardiologist, and if need be, the cardiologist refers to a surgeon, the best dentists refer patients with orthodontic needs to orthodontists. Orthodontists are required to take two to three extra years of university education beyond dental school and additional continuing clinical education every year. They must also invest in state-of-the-art technology for their offices (not found in dental offices) —*all for a good reason.*

Even though we orthodontists have the education and training to perform general dentist procedures, we don't. We specialize.

CHAPTER 5

How to Confidently Choose an Orthodontist

What are some good clues to selecting a great doctor?

I've got two: One, he's busy. His practice is busy.

I assure you, the ability of advertising to attract patients is limited and it's expensive. When you see a really, really busy practice, there are probably a whole lot of patient referrals, and neither kids or parents enthusiastically refer if they feel they were lied to or treated badly, put in pain or wound up with results nothing like the digital future-photo they were shown. And they probably wouldn't come to that practice if they had to keep coming back to "fix a few things," or were overcharged. Parents tell parents about great practices because we earned their trust and because their kids keep thanking them.

I keep my office very busy. Yes, we advertise. But mostly, these practices thrive by patient referrals. Not that I would anyway, but I don't need to goad you into more or more expensive care than your son's or daughter's situation requires for the best outcome. I don't need to "sell" four more sets of braces this month to win a cruise from the manufacturer—and yes, that stuff goes on in some practices. There's an old cartoon from The Wall Street Journal with a bunch of executives in a boardroom at a conference table, one hollering, "Ethics? Ethics? We can't afford ethics!"

This is a business, a business built on ethics and earned trust. And you do not just need a doctor to install braces; you need a trustworthy, trusted advisor.

The other clue: a great doctor is *not* cheap.

Our fees are calculated to allow for "Cadillac + Care" in every respect, to put no downward financial pressure on how we care for patients and parents, and to never cut corners or take shortcuts. We never use any material that is "probably good enough."

If I were you, I'd worry if I could find a doctor that is a lot cheaper anywhere else. If you do find one, know this: behind closed doors they're probably asking, "Can we do this cheaper?" Is that the question you want discussed back there, at every step of your child's treatment?

This isn't even like Botox. It's more like cosmetic surgery. There's a science and an art to this. My orthodontists and my staff are all highly trained to produce state-of-the-art outcomes, nothing less. The doctor makes a difference. That's why I tell everybody to get a highly successful doctor.

The Top Ten Things You Should Know *Before* Choosing Your Doctor

This is something you want to be sure about. I've just suggested one big consideration: a very successful practice. Here are ten more.

1. **Are they a specialist?**
   Orthodontists who are specially trained dentists who take on several extra years of training in order to "straighten teeth," usually by affixing braces to the patient's teeth. You might say we specialize in smiles.

   Orthodontists also perform dentofacial orthopedics. This is a fancy way to describe how we normalize the structure of a patient's jawbones in order to repair any imbalance in their face. All orthodontists are dentists, but only 6 percent of dentists are orthodontists. Look for the seal of the American Association of Orthodontists (AAO). Only orthodontic specialists can belong to the AAO.

2. **Do they treat adults?**
   Orthodontics is not just for kids! It's important that your orthodontist can treat patients of all ages. Many adults are finding out how a healthy and attractive smile is important to their health and the way they feel about themselves. Others choose to avoid a lifetime of crooked teeth for health concerns or problems with their bite.

3. **Do they provide the first visit free of charge?**
   Most orthodontists offer free examinations for new patients so you and your family can get expert advice about treatment needs, options, and timing before making this important investment. During your first exam and consultation be sure your questions are answered, your concerns are addressed, and you are educated about all of your treatment options. The orthodontist should include digital X-rays during the exam at no charge.

4. Do they offer guarantees? If so, what are they?

No matter which orthodontist you choose, ultimately you are not making a small investment. That being said, wouldn't you want to ensure your orthodontist is going to stand behind their treatment? Of course! At Bowen Orthodontics, we wouldn't have it any other way. In fact, we offer a satisfaction guarantee. If your child has any issues or if you are not satisfied with the treatment, our team of smile specialists will make it right, guaranteed.

5. Are they using the latest technology and treatment options available?

Orthodontics today differs a great deal from years past. Computer-designed braces and wires dramatically increase the precision with which we move teeth and shorten treatment time. Tie-free braces systems have made treatment far more efficient and comfortable.

Clear braces offer a cosmetically pleasing alternative, while Invisalign offers patients an entirely brace-free option. Did you know that Invisalign also has a special treatment system just for teens?

At Bowen Orthodontics, we can even place braces behind your teeth to make the entire treatment a well-kept secret! Ultimately, you get the best treatment available when you choose our office.

6. Does their quoted fee include retainers?

Each orthodontic office has its own fee schedules, and doctors often charge differently for procedures. All orthodontists should offer you a contract that clearly spells out the expenses for your child's treatment before it begins.

Throughout the orthodontic industry, it's common to find out about retainer fees after you start treatment. You should ask your orthodontist about what retainers cost and also if there are any other hidden fees.

7. Do they charge for emergency appointments?

Some minor discomfort may occur with braces. Orthodontists typically provide adjustments for poking wires and loose appliances free of charge.

At Bowen, we do provide these types of adjustments free of charge, but you should definitely ask about adjustments and potential costs with your orthodontist before you start treatment.

Keep in mind; if your braces are broken or damaged due to noncompliance with dietary restrictions, this may result in repair charges. With Bowen Orthodontics, if you do your best to avoid breaking your braces and follow the simple dietary guidelines that we will share with you, then you should have no additional costs for adjustments throughout your treatment, even if it's an emergency.

8. Do they make you feel special and comfortable?

Regardless if you are reading this book for your own treatment or for your child's treatment, when you meet with your orthodontist, you should definitely feel comfortable. At Bowen Orthodontics, we strive to make you as comfortable as possible before, during, and after treatment. You are special and we want you to feel special every time you see us.

Particularly important if you are reading this book for the treatment of your child, we also ensure your child feels special every time they visit. Since our doctors are so involved with children and young adults, we can empathize, relate to them, and make them feel comfortable and extra special.

9. Do they have a great reputation?

With the Internet, it is extremely easy to pull up ratings and reviews from patients. Simply go to Google and search for orthodontist reviews and ratings with your town.

Additionally, look on the website for video testimonials from actual patients. You can also ask the orthodontist for references.

Finally, you should make sure your orthodontist is a member of the Better Business Bureau and has a great rating with them. Being a member of the BBB shows you that the orthodontist takes pride in providing great customer service and treats patients the way they should be treated.

10. Are they flexible with payment options?

Once you are comfortable and you know specifically which orthodontist you want to treat you or your child, the next question is typically, "How much is this going to cost and how am I going to pay for this?" We help you understand different payment options from maximizing the most insurance benefits to flex spending accounts to even interest-free payment plans. During the initial exam and complimentary consultation, we will answer all of your questions, including those about our typical cost of braces and the variety of payment options available.

How to Know What Questions to Ask

I've really thought through the questions most parents and patients have—not just the ones they all ask but the ones they don't. This book attempts to cover them all, but overall, this is a *personal* matter. The best questions to ask are the ones that matter most to you and your child.

I hope not, but you may be in a position absolutely requiring you to get the minimum essential treatment for the lowest cost. If so, your most important questions are going to be about those kinds of options and about price, and about nothing else.

If, however, you are able to make your decision about who you should trust with your child's oral health and smile by many factors, we've included a "What Is Most Important to You?" quiz from Excellence In Orthodontics, on the following pages. As you'll see, there are fourteen different items to consider and rank in importance to you. Any can become the questions you ask me and my team or any other orthodontist.

If you have a specific question not answered anywhere in this book, or have a personal and confidential question, you can—with compete assurance of privacy and courtesy—call our office at any time to discuss you or your child's needs. There is also a FAQ section at the back of this book.

Of course, a perfect opportunity to get questions answered—yours and your son's or daughter's—is at your exam appointment.

Quiz: What Is Most Important to You?

Directions: For each Key Item below, rank its importance to you from 1 to 5. Then check off whether each type of provider provides that item. When you're done with all 14 Key Items, add up your rankings and review what your final score means about choosing an orthodontist.

Key Items to Consider in Selecting Your Orthodontist	Rank How Important Each Item Is To You in Selecting Your Orthodontist 1 - NOT Important, 5 - VERY Important	Check Off If Provided		
		Bowen Orthodontics	Other Provider	Other Provider
1 Orthodontist and staff committed to expert, thorough diagnosis and prescription of the best treatment plan customized for my son or daughter	1 2 3 4 5	✓		
2 Avoiding extractions (if possible)	1 2 3 4 5	✓		
3 Avoiding having to wear headgear with braces (if possible)	1 2 3 4 5	✓		
4 Avoiding "metal-mouth" braces (if possible) or utilizing the new type of "invisible" braces	1 2 3 4 5	✓		
5 Having a healthy, pleasing smile that will last a lifetime and protect optimum dental heath (not just having straightened teeth)	1 2 3 4 5	✓		
6 Pain-free treatment	1 2 3 4 5	✓		
7 Orthodontist utilizes the most modern, advanced, and proven technology, including computer-aided design and fitting	1 2 3 4 5	✓		
8 Orthodontists and team actively involved in continuing clinical education	1 2 3 4 5	✓		

Key Items to Consider in Selecting Your Orthodontist	Rank How Important Each Item Is To You in Selecting Your Orthodontist 1 - NOT Important, 5 - VERY Important	Check Off If Provided		
		Bowen Orthodontics	Other Provider	Other Provider
9 Reducing treatment time to a minimum without compromising results (including total length of treatment term and number of office visits)	1 2 3 4 5	✓		
10 Availability of after-school or after-work appointment options	1 2 3 4 5	✓		
11 Treatment Coordinator is knowledgeable about insurance coverage and is able to offer flexible payment plans	1 2 3 4 5	✓		
12 Getting the best overall value factoring in thorough diagnosis, customized care, and concern with lifetime health and well-being—not just the cheapest fee	1 2 3 4 5	✓		
13 Lifetime guarantee	1 2 3 4 5	✓		
14 Orthodontist and team committed to excellence in orthodontics and customer service for both patients and parents	1 2 3 4 5	✓		

Total of Your Rankings

What Your Score Means

50 to 70 There is no doubt. Bowen Orthodontics is the right choice for you and your family! It is clear that you place a high value on a comprehensive, "best" approach.

43 to 49 You are probably also going to be happiest with Bowen Orthodontics, rather than any other alternative. But this score suggests you aren't completely sure and have some unanswered questions or concerns. Your doctor and the practice's treatment coordinator want no lingering uncertainties on your part, and want to address any and every question. Don't keep anything to yourself. Please ask.

42 or less Frankly, you may not value the advanced, sophisticated level of clinical care and customer service provided at Bowen Orthodontics. Cost may be much more important to you than other factors, or very basic service may be all you feel you need. It's perfectly okay. If you choose to shop around, be sure to use this checklist in evaluating other options. Remember, you do want everything right the first time and you want error-free orthodontics at a minimum.

CHAPTER 6

What Can I Expect at the Initial Consultation and Exam?

Many questions surround your first visit to a new orthodontist, not the least of which is the subject of this particular chapter: *what will happen at the initial consultation?*

To answer this very common question, and perhaps several others you might not even realize you need answering yet, let me walk you through the typical first office visit, from the initial appointment forward. Your first appointment is scheduled following your initial phone call to your orthodontist's office

1: **On arrival at the office, you will be greeted by one of our certified treatment coordinators.** She or he is fully prepared to make everything from the first appointment to an entire treatment program go smoothly for you and your child. Your treatment coordinator will be yours, to manage your relationship with us, from appointment scheduling for your convenience to answering questions.

   At the initial visit, your treatment coordinator will review your child's patient information and health history and and/or any appearance concerns with you.

   This interview and required-by-law paperwork doesn't take long. You may also be asked to view, with your son or daughter, a pre-exam video by Excellence In Orthodontics. This video makes you and, if old enough, your son or daughter truly *informed* patients. It can reduce resistance by your preteen or teen to treatment, making life easier for you.

2: **Next, your orthodontist will conduct the "Customized Smile Analysis,"** the most complete and thorough orthodontic exam, including teeth, gums, mouth, jaws, and face. Typically, safe digital X-rays are taken of the teeth and surrounding bone and of the jaw structures. Molds of the teeth may be made.

Usually that same day, your orthodontist will present his or her "report of findings," a "show-n-tell" in plain English (not medical jargon) of the full state of your child's teeth, gums, mouth and jaws, and diagnosis of any present or anticipated problems that should get orthodontic treatment. If treatment should occur, your orthodontist will present recommendations and options. This will be an individualized, personalized plan of treatment, not "braces in a box, off the shelf." By this report of findings, you will know:

- What teeth or jaw misalignment or other problems exist or are developing

- What the health ramifications are of not intervening with treatment

- What the appearance ramifications are of not intervening with treatment

- If braces are needed now or later

- Which type of braces will be best in your situation

- What the complete treatment program will consist of: things like braces, number of appointments, and average time of each office visit

- What results will be achieved

3: **All your questions will be answered.** There are no dumb or embarrassing questions. Of the countless patients who have visited my office, every one of them had questions! We do not want you or your son or daughter just nodding, then later wondering, "what did he mean by that?" or saying "I wish I'd asked about ..." This is not one of those "I'm the doctor—trust me—just do what I say because I said so"offices. Most questions will have been answered by the pre-exam video, other literature provided to you, this book, and your orthodontist's report of findings, but it's a lot to take in. So, any and all questions you have should be asked and answered. Our goal is not just a terrific orthodontic outcome ensuring a healthy, attractive smile but also your anxiety-free comfort from start to finish.

4: Finally, your treatment coordinator will explain the costs of the prescribed treatment program and discuss payment arrangements as needed. Presuming proceeding, the next two appointments will be scheduled, for the installation of braces and/or other treatment. As the saying goes, a journey of a thousand steps begins with the first one, and a task well begun is sooner done!

In total, you should allow about one hour for this entire initial consultation and exam.

If that seems like a lot, keep in mind there are lifetime health, appearance, and personality aspects of this. And it is not "installing tires"—not if it is done properly and expertly. Your son or daughter deserves a careful, thorough, and anxieties-eliminated experience. You want to make the best decisions for them.

Frankly, our practice and our process is not for everybody. We attract and "resonate with" parents who are quite serious about their responsibilities and committed to giving their child every possible advantage in life—certainly not unnecessary disadvantages. If you are that parent, and the fact that you took the trouble to obtain and read this book suggests it, then you are going to recognize that this is time well invested in the best possible results.

Call us at 573-212-8723 or go to www.bowenortho.com to schedule your own Customized Smile Analysis.

CHAPTER 7

What Are the Treatment Options?

If your child is ready for orthodontic care, one of the first discussions to have with your orthodontist is which procedure is right for him or her; there might be more options than you had ever imagined.

If you're like most people, you associate orthodontists with braces, but these days that is just one arm of what I or any orthodontist does. Here are some of the services most orthodontists will provide their patients with during the course of routine treatment:

- Metal, tie-free braces
- Lingual braces placed behind your teeth
- Invisalign clear removable aligners
- Clear braces
- Expanders to match jaw size and tooth size
- Habit appliances to eliminate thumb sucking
- Space maintainers
- Retainers to prevent crowding and shifting of teeth
- Headgear to help correct jaw alignment
- Functional appliances to help improve facial balance
- Early treatment and growth modification
- Customized appliances designed uniquely for each patient

While many of these services may seem self-explanatory to you, several will probably not. In the following pages, I will try to elaborate on several of them, including:

- Crossbite correction
- Metal braces
- Clear braces
- Invisalign

Crossbite Correction

As your child's teeth begin to grow in, there's a lot more at work than mere gum lines, tooth fairies, and molar size. How the jaw is shaped, when it develops, and even how "normally" it develops can all affect the placement and comfort of your child's teeth.

When the upper and lower teeth grow at different rates, or even when the lower jaw grows disproportionately with the upper jaw, something known as a "crossbite" can occur.

Your child might have a crossbite if, for instance, the lower jaw is out of line with the upper jaw (kind of like a box that won't close right because one of the hinges is bent).

Or perhaps on the right side of your child's mouth, the lower teeth "stick out" a little farther than the top teeth, making the upper teeth on that side overlap in turn.

Or maybe your child's upper and lower jaws are out of alignment so instead of the top and bottom front teeth meeting "naturally" as they should, the front teeth fall somewhat behind the lower teeth. This would be the reverse of an overbite.

As you might imagine, any or all of these developments can lead to short- and long-term discomfort for your child.

How, When, and Why Crossbites Form

You might be amazed to find out how many ways a crossbite can form as your child grows and develops during his or her formative years. Heredity is one key to jaw growth, or alignment, as is the size of your child's developing jaw.

Another factor that can contribute to the development of a potential crossbite is if it takes your child too long to lose his or her baby teeth. In some extreme cases, in fact, if it takes too long for your child to lose his baby teeth, another set of teeth can grow in behind them, throwing the alignment off and contributing to a crossbite.

Believe it or not, something as basic as whether your child breathes through her nose or her mouth can also contribute to a crossbite. While most children breathe through their noses, some children develop a habit early on of breathing through their mouths instead.

In children who breathe through their noses while they're sleeping, the tongue naturally rests on the roof of the mouth, promoting natural and proper upper jaw growth. When young children breathe through their mouths, however, the tongue relocates from the roof of the mouth to the bottom, removing that extra support and potentially contributing to reduced upper jaw bone growth; this can create the crossbite we spoke of previously.

How Can I Spot a Crossbite?

Although it sounds severe, and even painful from the description provide earlier, the effects of a crossbite can take time to manifest themselves. Still, here are some of the telltale signs your child might be cultivating, or already suffering from, a crossbite:

- Snoring
- Difficulty breathing
- Chewing on one side of the mouth or the other
- Signs of an underbite
- If your child's chin seems "off center" or disproportionate

How, When, and Why to Correct a Crossbite

Where should you start looking for treatment if you're concerned about your child's jaw development after reading this section? If you suspect your child might have a crossbite, approach your family dentist about a recommendation for a specialist such as an orthodontist.

There are many possible treatments available for a crossbite, and your orthodontist can work with you closely to make the right and specific decisions for you and your child.

When should you start? I believe you know my standard answer when it comes to questions like this one: *as early as possible!* The same way an auto mechanic would tell you to take care of that oil leak, bulging tire, or faulty timing belt sooner rather than later, myself and my colleagues in orthodontics will always favor early treatment to later.

Crossbites are often closely linked with other orthodontic issues, such as teeth alignment, jaw size, and growth, so naturally, the sooner you address any or all of these issues, the better.

Finally, why should you address a crossbite? Crossbites can lead to pain, discomfort, and a lack of confidence as your child begins to feel insecure or even ostracized because of this very treatable, very normal series of jaw and teeth developments.

Not only can crossbites become physically uncomfortable if left untreated, but if the misalignment or root cause of the bite isn't fixed early in childhood, then the child's appearance and, ultimately, confidence could be affected as the crossbite becomes more pronounced in adolescence.

Metal Braces

The fact is, metal braces still have a valued place in the orthodontic world, and despite advances and breakthroughs of products like Invisalign and even clear braces, they aren't going extinct anytime soon! This is because metal braces are very strong and can withstand most types of treatment. Today's metal braces are smaller, sleeker, and more polished than ever before.

Older, traditional metal braces require an elastic o-shaped rubber band, called a ligature, to hold the arch wire onto the bracket. These elastic ties collect more plaque and bacteria, making it harder for patients to clean the teeth and gums.

You may have heard of "speed braces." These are sometimes also referred to as "self-ligating brackets" or "tie-free braces." Self-ligating means that the brackets do not need the little o-shaped rubber bands (ligatures) or metal tie wires to hold the arch wire onto the bracket. Several companies have developed braces for holding the wires in place without ligatures.

By using self-ligation technology, the brackets allow the wire to slide back and forth. This advancement allows for fewer adjustments and fewer appointments. These types of braces do not need rubber bands to hold the arch wire in place. They use a "door" to secure the arch wire to the bracket. They're smaller than traditional metal and less food gets trapped around them when you eat.

Your orthodontist might use an advanced self-ligating bracket that does not require physical tightening of the wire to the braces. It's a twin bracket made of metal or clear ceramic and utilizes a special built-in clip. The pressure from specific types of arch wires activates the clip and delivers specific amounts of force to each tooth, resulting in fast, directed results.

Naturally, orthodontists are very excited about the hygiene benefits of these self-closing or tie-free metal braces. Patients are excited that their braces are small, smooth, and friction-free and straighten their teeth in fewer visits with less discomfort than braces with wires that are "tied-in."

Clear Braces

Ceramic braces are very strong and generally do not stain. Two popular brands are Clarity, made by 3M Unitek, and Empower, made by American Orthodontics. Adults like to choose ceramic because they "blend in" with the teeth and are less noticeable than metal. These are the type of braces actor Tom Cruise had.

Older types of ceramic braces required white or clear ligatures (tiny rubber bands) to hold the wire on to the braces. Empower is a revolutionary tie-free ceramic braces system that combines the same efficient tooth movement with exceptional aesthetics. Patients choosing Empower no longer have to decide between metal braces or clear braces that could stain.

Today's clear Empower braces are very aesthetic because they no longer require the small rubber bands that could stain with certain foods or drinks.

Adult Orthodontics

It's not uncommon for individuals who have undergone orthodontic treatment earlier in life to find their teeth have drifted out of alignment over the years. Most adults won't think twice about bleaching their teeth to roll back the effects of time. Yet few think about the role orthodontics can play.

Adults of all ages can enjoy the same cosmetic and health benefits of properly aligned teeth with appliances like the Empower system braces.

Improperly aligned teeth can do more than undermine your confidence. They can make proper cleaning and brushing more difficult, contribute to enamel loss and even set the stage for more significant problems down the road. Fortunately, discrete treatment with Empower braces can help keep you aligned with a healthy, happy lifestyle.

The Solution Is *Clear*

Orthodontists believe every individual has the right to live their life with a smile they truly love, particularly children. Healthy, straight, and attractive smiles make your child happier and more self-confident. And isn't that what we all want for them?

Empower helps you achieve the smile of your dreams faster, easier, and more discretely than you ever imagined. Embrace the confidence that comes with beautifully aligned teeth and put your smile on display. Schedule a consultation and ask if Empower system braces are right for you.

The Empower system uses a free-sliding technology that places almost no pressure on your teeth as it gently corrects their alignment. Less pressure means a more comfortable treatment.

With Empower free-sliding braces, your treatment can proceed faster with fewer follow-up visits than traditional fixed wire braces.

Invisalign

Invisalign is a widely advertised, well-known, and popular braces product, and often, kids know about it and ask parents and doctors for it by name. For many, it's as good an option as any other and sometimes even the best option.

Invisalign uses advanced, proprietary 3-D computer imaging technology to "map" the entire span of treatment, from the present teeth alignment to the desired positioning, alignment, and smile. Clear aligners are custom made and based on the 3-D imaging. Invisalign has many features that have helped make it such a popular choice. The aligners are removable, even before a snack or meal as well as for general hygiene. There are no metal brackets or wires. Office visits for adjustments throughout the treatment program are fast, easy and painless. The thermoplastic aligners are virtually invisible. Over one million patients have been treated with Invisalign, and there is a special Invisalign system for teens.

Because Invisalign is computer mapped, there's sometimes the idea that anybody can install Invisalign and that all practitioners using Invisalign are the same. I have an important warning about this: during each stage of the complete treatment, only certain teeth are allowed to move. Which teeth move in what order, and the amount of time (days/weeks) needed for each successive set of aligners differs for each patient. *This* is what you rely on an expert orthodontist specializing in pediatric and juvenile care to decide. At the start, we determine whether your son or daughter is a good candidate for the Invisalign approach, or if they would be better served with different braces. You have to rely on *somebody* to tell you. I promise you, there are kids who've been hurried to Invisalign who were not good candidates for it.

Invisalign Teen

Much like the standard adult version, the Invisalign Teen System lets you do it the modern, hygienic way. Your new smile is created with the most innovative technology—a series of clear aligners that are custom-fit to your teeth.

The first thing you should know is that an average treatment takes about a year. Plus, your treatment can begin even if you don't have all of your permanent teeth. Invisalign Teen was designed to meet your needs.

Invisalign Teen aligners will snap on your child's teeth easily. They are comfortable and practically invisible. Invisalign Teen allows for permanent teeth to grow gently and continuously moves teeth in small increments. Aligners are worn for about two weeks and then swapped for a new pair.

Invisalign Teen aligners have a "Blue Dot Wear Indicator," designed to show an estimation of wear time. The dot is designed to fade until it's clear over a two-week period if you wear your aligners properly (meaning for 20 to 22 hours every day).

Invisalign Teen is designed to custom-fit to your child's teeth and go with his or her lifestyle. During your treatment, your child can keep smiling, playing sports, eating what he or she wants, and brushing and flossing normally. Plus, unlike traditional braces, the aligners are made of smooth plastic and move teeth gradually.

The aligners can be removed for eating, brushing, and flossing or going to a special event. The aligners are replaceable if lost. That's right; you get up to six free individual aligners.

After your child's Invisalign Teen treatment, you may find his or her self-confidence boosted by their new smile and the change in their appearance. Some people even feel that way during the treatment. As you know, smiling has many benefits. It can help your child make a strong impression in lots of different social situations—at school, at work, or at a party.

Invisalign Teen really works. It helps correct a broad range of dental and orthodontic issues. You can get a confident smile without metal bands, brackets, or wires. It works on many kinds of conditions, including overly crowded or widely spaced teeth, crossbites, overbites, and underbites.

We've used Invisalign to successfully transform the smiles of many patients, but we do not prescribe it to everybody. After all, *popularity* should not govern medical care!

Trustworthy, Objective Advice

Bowen Orthodontics is *not* "in the pocket of" or obligated to any of these providers of different braces products and technologies. We select and recommend what we believe is the most appropriate and beneficial choice for your child. We are happy to discuss the pros and cons of different ones, if your child has heart set on, say, Invisalign, because that's what a friend has, or based on information you've obtained.

Candidly, these manufacturers vary in price to the orthodontist (or dentist) based on volume purchase benchmarks, incentivizing concentration of as much use as possible to one product. Awards are given out to the highest volume buyers and users. It's borderline unseemly. It introduces temptation into the diagnostic and prescriptive process, and I never let us bow to such incentives and temptations. The number-one rule here is: what is absolutely best for the patient?

CHAPTER 8

Will My Child Need Any Adult Teeth Removed?

Many parents wonder if their child will have to have any teeth removed. Many of them had them removed as a child and have assumed that technology has advances since then and their child won't have to have any teeth removed. For some parents, when they are told that their child will require adult teeth removed in order to have orthodontic treatment, it's a NO GO for them. Whether it is a fear of pain or discomfort for their child, a bad experience they had with tooth removal as a child, or just a sense that they "just don't want to" the thought of having to remove adult teeth makes them uneasy.

Here's the real scoop.

Most orthdontists (including me) would prefer not to remove adult teeth.

The orthodontic technology has advanced sincy the 1960's and 1970's to make treatment more comfortable and efficient, but no appliance or technology to day can over come biology

When absolutely indicated, sometimes removal of adult teeth is indicated.

My personal mission is to objectively help parents clearly understand why or why not removal of teeth is or isn't indicated. I help show how unattractive smiles and faces can be if teeth are not removed when indicated. Not to mention severe gum and bone loss in the future could result from NOT doing so(in cases where removal of teeth is indicated) Whoever you choose as your orthodontist should also have the same compassion and these same objectives.

Some orthodontists play into this parental fear of removing teeth and will claim that they NEVER remove teeth. They say the removal of teeth is "old-fashioned" treatment or claim that the types of braces/ techniques they use are "special" and avoid having to remove teeth. One of the latest claims on the internet suggests that removing teeth will lead to any one of a number of chronic conditions as an adult, including TMD and sleep apnea.

All of these claims are not only false, but are simple marketing pitches from companies and orthodontists so their businesses can financially benefit, regardless of any actual benefit to you child. These sentiments are also extremely dangerous and irresponsible, as this means the orthodontist is looking at cramming all the teeth in as the sole objective. This comes with a lack of understanding of the role of other structures of you child's face and bite as part of the big picture.

I only suggest tooth removal when all other methods to avoid to avoid doing so are exhausted, and when it's objectively in your child's best interest. The orthodontist you ultimately choose for you family should also feel the same way.

The bottom-line is that you, as a parent, have to feel comfortable and clearly know the reasons why tooth removal is or is not indicated. Your orthodontist should adequately, and objectively explain why or why not you child would benefit from either decision and you should feel comfortable with their recommendation. If you do not, by all means then you SHOULD seek a second opinion!

CHAPTER 9

How to Pay for Orthodontic Treatment & Braces

You may have never needed braces. Or you may have needed them and gotten them. Or you may be among the tens of thousands of people in our generation who needed them but did not get them, perhaps because your family decided they couldn't afford them. Maybe they didn't consider it a priority and probably underestimated the lifelong results of the decision. You may not only have lived with a "hide your smile" habit unnecessarily, but you may have developed chronic jaw pain and headaches, difficulty chewing, or even periodontal disease that could have been prevented.

Regardless of which group you're in—and I hope it's not the third—I hope you will be making the best choices for your son or daughter today, without being hamstrung just by the finances. Truth is, parents pay out the same cost for a number of different things not nearly as vital as health or emotional well-being without blinking, mostly because it's paid in installments or just never really *considered,* like the monthly cost for minutes/data on mobile devices, added up for a year or two. The additional insurance cost and other costs when the teenager gets his driver's permit; after all, what's the choice? The cost of braces leaps up and stands there, all at one time. So it can seem big. And it tempts thoughts of "maybe later" or "is this really necessary?"

I hope in the prior chapters I have succeeded at getting the "is it really necessary?" question erased. If there is visible need or if expert examination by an orthodontist and his explanation of what he finds and can show you say it is advisable, it is necessary! It won't fix itself. It will probably get worse. It plagues a person's health, emotional well-being, social life, and career. It can link to very serious medical problems. *Necessary* is not really debatable.

Now let's tackle the ugly matter of the money.

I say "ugly" because nobody really likes talking about this. Most orthodontists are nervous about it. Parents are uncomfortable with it. If there is a financial obstacle to treatment, most people are reluctant to admit it, offer other excuses, and then can't be helped by the doctor. I think we have to trust each other. With me, this discussion is entirely confidential, in a "safe zone." Orthodontists are not Martians, by the way; we have kids, college tuitions that loom, and family budgets.

What Is a Reasonable Fee and Cost?

A complete treatment program, including braces, can cost anywhere from $4,000 to $10,000 or so. Most fall in between. Adjusted for inflation, these prices are actually *less than* braces decades ago, while the technology and quality has advanced. In costs it can prevent later, it's a bona fide bargain. TMJ treatments are expensive. Cosmetic dentistry work is expensive. Migraine headache drugs are expensive and have side effects.

For this investment, you will be getting the carefully selected, personalized solution to your child's irregularities and problems, prescribed using state-of-the-art digital technology along with the expertise of a specialist, and considerate, compassionate care from start to finish. Your investment includes a varying number of appointments plus the orthodontic appliance itself, after-care, and in my office, certain guarantees.

It's hard to really draw a fair comparison, but if you have any significant net worth, you can easily pay similar fees for the services of an attorney expert in estate planning. Most kitchen remodels cost considerably more. Where real expertise is involved and the stakes of getting it wrong are high, you can't escape professional level fees.

In this case, the $4,000 to $10,000 range is seen as perfectly reasonable by the overwhelming majority of parents that I talk to. Each year, we provide braces of one kind or another to countless patients. Even parents who shook their heads at the cost to start with tell me afterward that having witnessed everything we do to get the absolute best obtainable results, and seeing the outcome itself, they feel undercharged.

While it's never easy to part with such a sum, people do it every day for all sorts of less important things, and when they do often pay for something like their new designer handbag, golf vacation, or suite of living room furniture. They'll pay for it outright or with their favorite credit card (getting the reward points in the bargain). If you put the orthodontic treatment program including braces on a typical credit card at the interest in play as I write this, and you choose to make only the minimum required monthly payment, your monthly payments will be relatively small. Even tight budgets can accommodate this *when it is really important.* It's less than most families pay for their cable and streaming entertainment. For many, if they got all their Starbucks stops consolidated into one monthly bill, it would be more than this!

Health Spending Accounts (HSA) /Flex Spending Accounts (FSA)

The HSA allows you to set aside pre-tax dollars to be used for certain medical and health expenses for you or your family. They exist although restricted under the Affordable Care Act (Obamacare) as it stood in July of 2017. By the time you read this, the opportunity may have been expanded, as President Trump suggested. In any case, if you have accumulated money in an HSA, you can probably spend it on orthodontic treatment. If you don't have an HSA, you might want to start one. Information can be found online about existing or new accounts and their rules of use, at www.healthcare.gov.

Other kinds of FSAs are typically set up through your place of employment and similarly enable you to set aside pre-tax dollars for medical expenses. Sometimes, employers match contributions. Again, you can almost certainly tap funds from your FSA for your child's orthodontic care. Check with your employer about this.

If you have a tax accountant, you may want to consult with him about your HSA or FSA.

TIP: *How can you make the most out of your employer's flex-pay plan?*

First, make sure you understand how it works. Second, set aside flex-spending dollars in advance of need, and if possible, make the maximum contributions. Many employers allow higher limits than you'd think without asking, as much as $2,500 to $5,000 per year. Be aware of "family status changes" allowed by your plan that may enable you to change the amount being moved pre-tax from your paychecks to your account anytime during the year rather than just once at the first of the year—so you could bump up the amount in months before the first orthodontic treatment. IMPORTANT: Be aware of the balance and the loss of unused funds. In most cases, if you do not use these funds, you lose them, year to year. You usually have three months after the end of the calendar year to submit claims for eligible expenses from the previous year.

Insurance

These days, there are as many different types of insurance plans as there are patients in my office. I can't possibly speak to your unique and personal insurance policy without seeing it first but, in general, my experience tells me that "most" insurance policies cover "some" of your orthodontic expenses.

I realize that answer sounds very vague, but here are a couple of variables you need to answer before an insurance agent can help you determine what, how long, and how many procedures fall under your insurance:

- The type of procedure (braces, Invisalign, etc.)
- The duration of the procedure (two months, six months, a year, etc.)
- The cause of the procedure (a patient presenting with pain, a parent's concern, traumatic injury or accident, congenital birth defect like cleft lip or palate etc.)
- The nature of the procedure (to correct pain/discomfort, cosmetic, etc.)

I can only partially answer this question, but talking to your insurance agent will help you get the right answers you need.

> **TIP: Keep an insurance journal of every interaction with your carrier.**
>
> Write down the date, time of call, name of the person you contacted, and the exact instructions or recommendations following the call.
>
> Later, if your insurance company doesn't remember what they told you, you'll have it accurately written down. If they still don't remember, ask them to pull the recorded audio tape from your previous call, so that you can accurately "remind" them of exactly what they told you.

Loans

If you qualify, we offer Lending Point, which can provide an unsecured, signature-only loan for the treatment program, with repayment over twelve to sixty months. You don't need to go anywhere else to apply or do paperwork; we can take care of it in my office.

If you have equity in your home, the lowest-cost loan option may be a home equity line of credit or second mortgage. See your own bank, or check out RocketMortgage at rocket.quickenloans.com. As of this writing, mortgage interest is at record lows.

Obviously, a private loan from a family member can be the easiest option. A lot of preteens' and teens' important orthodontic care is financed at the Bank of Grandma and Grandpa.

If the other options are difficult or unavailable, we will set up a weekly, bimonthly, or monthly "paycheck payment plan" with a comfortable monthly payment.

What If You Really, Really Can't Afford Braces?

I have compiled a list of eighteen ways you may be able to substantially reduce the cost of braces. Frankly, some of them are less than ideal, and most are not available through my office, but they could be helpful if your back is really up against a financial wall.

1. **Get braces in April or November and see if you can save a little extra by paying in full.** These are the months that orthodontists are the least-busy, and it's when we have our most meetings (April–May). In November, everyone is getting ready for the holidays or the office is closed the week of Thanksgiving. By scheduling during the "off season," you can often find better deals with willing orthodontists.

2. **See if you can get a discount for not breaking any brackets.** Believe it or not, most orthodontists would happily take $100 off your final bill if you don't break any appliances throughout treatment!

3. **New technology; better pricing.** See if you can be one of your orthodontist's first patients with a new technology and save some money on the lab fee or receive a discount for being a teaching case.

4. **See if your local dental school has an orthodontic program.** The treatment at such institutions is supervised by board-certified orthodontists (most of whom practice in the surrounding area). While you might spend a little more time in

the chair as a teaching case, if you have the time, it might be well worth the wait because you can save up to half the cost of traditional braces.

5. **Ask your insurance plans when they send out their fee schedules to participating providers.** If the insurance company updates their fees or the orthodontist raises his or her fees to keep up with the cost of inflation, it might be around November in preparation for the next year.

6. **See your dentist every four to six months.** While you're wearing your braces, the extra cleaning each year can prevent tooth decay, a costly item to repair.

7. **Get your flex spending dollars in order with your employer.** If you set money aside in a flex plan, it may be "tax-free" but it comes with some stipulations: namely, you have to use it before the end of the year or else you lose it.

8. **See if you can get a second set of retainers from your orthodontist at the end of treatment.** Sometimes getting two sets of retainers at the same time can be cheaper than buying a second set later in life when you lose or break your first set.

9. **See if your husband or wife has an insurance plan that covers braces.** Be sure to enroll in the plan with enough time to spare before your child needs braces, so that the procedure is not denied by your insurance company due to a waiting period.

10. **Ask for flexible financing options.** When you boil it down to the basics, your orthodontist really just wants to help you. Regardless of his specialty, your doctor spent way too much time in school not to love what he does. If you're easy to work with, keep your teeth clean and avoid breaking your braces while you're wearing them, he or she will probably be thrilled to help you finance the care, or find another way to afford the investment.

11. **Do you have multiple kids in treatment?** If so, take advantage of that fact and see if you can get a family discount.

12. **If finances are extremely tight, you should check out the organizations that orthodontists have created to help provide pro-bono care, such as SmilesChangeLives.org.** There are even more foundations like this if you have a cleft palate or other facial anomalies, like the Rheam Foundation for Cleft and Craniofacial Research.

13. **School auctions, churches, or public service entities will often receive donations from local orthodontists wishing to donate a case to the school or organization for a fundraiser.** Checking around local school newsletters or church bulletins for their upcoming silent auctions could be a great find! If you're unwilling to leave such things to chance, call your local schools or churches and ask them specifically if they have such a fund and, if so, how to apply/qualify.

14. **If you're thinking about a career change, apply at your local orthodontist's office.** Most orthodontists offer free braces to their staff and their children as an employee benefit! (And you never know, you could love your career and your child's new braces!)

15. **Military, schoolteachers and firefighters sometimes receive special courtesies in dental and orthodontic offices throughout the year.** Keep your ears open and you might save a few bucks or at least get a donation from the orthodontist to your organization.

16. **This tactic won't save you any money, but it could earn your organization or business some money if you have a newsletter, sports team, fund-raiser, or special event that needs a sponsor.** Ask your orthodontist. Most orthodontic offices are huge supporters of the communities in which they practice and would probably love to advertise with your organization.

17. **Got taxes?** Good! Why not use your tax refund to help pay for treatment in full and ask for a courtesy on the average fees associated with financing a full orthodontic case? In some areas, you can save as much as 10 percent on the cost of braces by simply saving your pennies and paying the entire bill at once, up front.

18. **Ask for more flexible financing, through a third-party credit company like Chase Healthcare Advance, through Lending Point, or by using in-house financing through your orthodontist.** Most orthodontists will accept a reasonable down payment and split the remaining amount into easy monthly payments for your convenience. With automated withdrawals from a checking or savings account, you might be able to stretch the monthly payments out over a longer period to make each payment lower. Just don't be shocked if your orthodontist asks you to approve a credit check. A little homework up front can be well worth the effort when your monthly orthodontic bill is lower than your cell phone bill!

There's no doubt about it; braces can be expensive. However, now that you're armed with these eighteen massive, budget-saving tips, you won't need to decide between braces and your budget ever again!

CHAPTER 10

Life with Braces

Remember, this *isn't* 1982. Or 1992. Today's braces aren't anything like yours if you had them decades ago. Today's orthodontic care is far more advanced, more sophisticated, and more patient-centered than any prior generation has experienced. If you had traditional metal braces twenty years or so ago, you experienced medieval torture. The dungeon is gone too, replaced by ultra-modern, patient comfort friendly offices. Out of the dark, into the light!

Living with braces is not going to be anywhere near as difficult as you might imagine.

Let's look at a few specific concerns.

Brushing and Hygiene

Modern braces, whether they're metal, flexible, or "invisible," are all actually made to fit the individual and facilitate easy, painless, thorough brushing. This means your child brushes pretty much the same as he would if he didn't have braces.

Here are some simple tips you can share with your child for the best results when brushing with braces on:

- Brush your teeth with a medium nylon toothbrush after you eat and before bed (no electric toothbrushes).*
- Brush, rinse, and look; if you find any areas that are not clean, brush them again.
- Brush your gums as you brush your teeth (massage and stimulate).
- Take extra care in the area between the gums and the braces, because food caught and left there can cause swollen gums, cavities, discomfort, and permanent teeth stains.
- If no toothpaste is available, brush without.
- If you are unable to brush, rinse your mouth vigorously with water.
- Replace your old toothbrush when it gets worn out.
- It's absolutely essential you continue regular visits to your family dentist for checkups and cleanings throughout your orthodontic treatment!

---

* At my office, you'll be provided with a home kit including the best toothbrush, toothpaste, and rinse.

Depending on the age of your child, you, the parent, may need to supervise the first few brushings with the braces in place. You should not have a whining, resistant, difficult child on your hands because of any of this. It should be painless, simple, and routine.

Forbidden Foods Your Child Must Avoid

After your child's orthodontic appliance/braces have been placed, the teeth are usually "tender" and sensitive for as few as three to as many as ten days: a *short* time. During these few days, softer foods are recommended: soups, macaroni, spaghetti, eggs, fish, Jell-O, yogurt. As needed, Tylenol or Advil are adequate in relieving any discomfort, taken an hour or so before eating.* Warm saltwater rinses can be helpful. We also provide a "soft white wax," a safe topical that eases gum discomfort.

For the entire duration of the braces being in place, I'd advise you to stay away from hard and sticky foods that can damage braces and may lengthen the time they have to be worn or even require extra office visits. Sugar-rich foods can make hygiene harder and cause calculus build-up and cavities. You're probably already monitoring and limiting your child's intake of such foods, so there's really nothing new under the sun here. But, for the record, here are the "featured items" that should be avoided during orthodontic treatment and wearing of braces:

1. **Rock-hard foods:** Ice (don't chew ice!), nuts, popcorn (has hard kernels inside), peanut brittle, rock candy, whole apples and carrots (unless cut into bite sized pieces), corn on the cob, hard pretzels, hard rolls, hard taco shells.
2. **Extra-sticky foods:** Jolly Ranchers or Starbursts or similar candies, bubble gum, taffy, and sticky Cinnabon rolls.
3. **Very chewy foods:** Pizza crust, beef jerky, gummy bears. Note: no chewing on pencils or pens.
4. **Super-sugary foods and drinks:** Soda pop with sugar, ice cream, most cookies and cake. Yes, this is the worst of the forbidden foods. Some kids will give you a tough time. But there are sugar-free versions of all these kinds of foods, to be made or baked, or store-bought.

---

* Prescription pain pills with dangerous side effects are not needed. Any orthodontist or dentist easily prescribing such drugs is not to be trusted. As you are no doubt aware from the news, opioid addiction is rampant. Pain drugs are, contrary to early assertions by their manufacturers, proving to be extremely addictive, for many people after nominal and legitimate use. I can't emphasize enough—we practice truly pain-free orthodontics.

We will speak about this with your son or daughter and give them a printed list, but you will have to reinforce, monitor, and provide some substitute foods to prevent mutiny or months of sulking. Most kids get it, though. When they understand how short or long the number of weeks of wearing braces will turn out to be, how comfortable or uncomfortable wearing them and hygiene while wearing them is, and how successful the outcome will be is linked to their staying away from the short list of harmful foods, they are pretty responsible about it.

Most parents who are initially really worried about this tell us later it wasn't the horror show they'd imagined.

Emergencies, Injuries, Travel, and Time Away from Home

Many "emergencies" actually aren't and can be easily and safely remedied at home. You are provided with a "What to Do in Case of the 5 Common Emergencies" printed card, and you can always access the same information at our web site, 24/7/365.

Common emergencies include the breaking of some part of the braces, eating something particularly damaging—even a McDonalds bun full of sesame seeds might feel like an emergency, or, early, a feeling of discomfort that worries something serious might be wrong. These are the sort of things addressed in the "What to Do" instructions.

If you do run up against an emergency that isn't easily managed with these instructions or can't wait for regular office hours, we have a special phone number to call that routes to a knowledgeable staff member directly or with return call within sixty minutes or less. All VIP Plan patients are guaranteed an office visit if needed, same day, seven days a week. You are never left out to dry.

If your family or son or daughter are away from home and say, they chomp down on a piece of toffee and break a piece of their braces, there is *always* a remedy. You are *not* going to cut your vacation short and rush to the airport! Again, often a remedy you do by our instructions can meet the urgent need until everybody gets back home. With some types of braces, we can FedEx temporary replacements. I also belong to a network of orthodontists with offices throughout the United States, which we can utilize in the *extremely rare instance* when getting to an orthodontist immediately is vital.

Here is just how good the appliances themselves and our management of orthodontic treatment has gotten. In 2016 to 2017:

Ninety-eight percent of patients required no extra office visits for repairs, adjustments, care or emergencies (beyond regularly scheduled office visits per their treatment plan).

Eighty-five percent called with questions, worries, or emergencies that were handled simply by advice and home remedy and/or waited without harm until the next regularly scheduled visit.

Sports

Speaking of injuries, the question of sports versus braces worries kids and parents alike. These days, kids are *very* active in organized and school sports, some starting one as another's season is ending. You know this; you are coordinating the schedules and working as their unpaid chauffeur.

Good news: for every sport and every level of play, there is either an inexpensive off-the-shelf mouth guard or a slightly costlier, custom-fit mouth guard to provide an extra, suitable level of dental protection and to protect the braces themselves. In some sports, additional face masks or other equipment normally treated as an option can be added and used during the time period of the orthodontic treatment. Ask us for guidance for your child and their sport(s). Some mouth guards even come with insurance against dental injury, covering financial costs.

We have thought this through! For example, research reported in Clinics in Sports Medicine, from the Department of Neurology at Boston University School of Medicine examined uses of different kinds of mouth guards and the rate of sports-related concussions. There was no significant difference in concussion risks found tied to different types of mouth guards. We can select the best one for your child, his sport and level of play and, if a factor, your budget with no worry about one choice instead of another affecting risk of concussion.

This, by the way, is typical of a good orthodontic specialist: attention to every detail. They should have a good knowledge of every ramification of wearing braces, clinical and technological advancements, and every patient or parent need. To be blunt, it's a practical impossibility for a general dentist to give the braces work he does on the side anywhere near this same level of all in focus.

By the way, there are collegiate and pro athletes, even NFL players, getting orthodontic treatment and even wearing braces. If they can, your child can! You do *not* need the drama of stopping your child from playing the sports they're committed to because of their orthodontic treatment. Oh, and we even guarantee your office visits will not cause you to miss work or business responsibilities, nor cause your child to miss school or organized sports.

See, this *isn't* going to be difficult!

Tips for Helping Your Child Adjust to a Life with Braces

- **All the cool kids are doing it (or soon will be):** Braces are a very popular appliance during the middle school and high school years. Rather than focus on how he or she feels wearing braces, encourage your child to begin actively looking for other kids who are wearing braces. Chances are, they'll find lots more than they ever imagined!

- **Even famous people do it:** Gwen Stefani. Prince Harry. Drew Barrymore. Tom Cruise. Dakota Fanning. Danny Glover. The list of famous people who've worn braces—many of them as adults—could fill half this book. Share with your child how even the most famous people in the spotlight sometimes need a little help through braces.

- **Fast forward:** Many orthodontists provide a "before and after" consultant's session, much like a plastic surgeon. Digital pictures are often used to portray what the child's teeth might look like once the braces have been removed. Have your child focus on the "after" when he or she gets down about the "before" shots!

- **Be prepared:** Finally, create a "master list" of things your child likes to do: things that make him feel special, confident, brave, calm, relaxed, or excited. If you notice him feeling down, consult your list and make plans to do something special in the near future to boost his confidence level back to where you know it belongs!

CHAPTER 11

Life After Braces: Retainers

So, your child's braces are off and they're ready to live a life full of confidence and good oral health. They may think, *I'm free! I'm free!* Well, not quite yet.

The selection of the right braces, the expert orthodontist, and the compliant wearing of the braces gets us about three-fourths of the way to where we want to be: a well-aligned, as-perfect-as-possible, healthy smile for life.

But after braces, there are retainers.

While many patients are understandably eager to be done with braces once they come off, the fact is, retainers do as much work—if not more—than the braces themselves. Straight teeth in proper alignment have to stay that way, and for that, retainers are a big help.

When the braces are removed, teeth can still shift if not helped through a period of adjustment, to settle in. Retainers gently but purposefully remind the teeth to stay straight during this adjustment period. It's advised that nearly all patients who've gone through the time, work, and expense of braces will want to use fixed or removable retainers for months or years or even for life and continue to schedule regular orthodontic check-ups. Some dentists doing braces won't tell you this, but I will. Years ago, clinicians believed that once teeth were straightened by braces, they would simply stay that way forever. New science says otherwise. In fact, teeth position shifting as we age is to be expected. Teeth naturally shift to the middle and crowd. So, retainers are actually extremely important in maintaining the new smile from braces.

Any claims otherwise, by some "brand" of braces or any doctor, are flat-out false.

Retainers can play a role in:

- Closing any gaps that may remain in the bite
- Correcting any speech problems—sometimes occurring with a new bite or jaw position

- Tongue thrust—where the tongue slips under the teeth while talking
- Bruxism—grinding teeth while sleeping

As you can see, there's a lot more to this than just "installing and removing braces."

In post-braces monitoring and check-ups, I tend to decide on the best kind of retainer for your child before the removal of the braces. Growth of the jaw following treatment (yes, the jaw is still growing in adolescents, to age eighteen or so), stabilizing of the gums and bone tissues, pressures from lips and tongue, and other factors tell me what type of retainer should be worn and for how long. Retainers are made out of rubber, plastic, and sometimes, still metal. They are custom made and fit, as part of the complete orthodontic treatment. However, after the initial orthodontic exam, at the same time the best braces are being selected, it's usually possible, with a good degree of certainty, to predict the type of retainer(s) your child is going to need, and I'm happy to share that information with you at that time.

Some retainers are invisible or nearly invisible. There are clear plastic retainers. A *fixed* retainer is typically placed on the inside/back surfaces of the lower front teeth. A fixed retainer may be used until lower jaw growth is complete and then no longer needed. When your child hears "retainer" he will most likely picture a *removable* retainer. These make hygiene easy, are easily removed and cleaned daily and can be removed for a sports activity.

There are even "fashion retainers" now—popular with kids of different ages—in school colors, and some even with pictures on them! In my office, patients using different kinds of retainers also receive clear, flexible plastic retainers as a back-up in case of damage to the main retainer or for occasional social functions where the preteen or teen "just can't be caught dead with a retainer in her mouth."

This is an important part of braces aftercare and part of the complete orthodontic treatment program personalized for your child.

Call us at 573-212-8723 or go to www.bowenortho.com to schedule your own Customized Smile Analysis.

CHAPTER 12

Life After Braces: Wisdom Teeth

I hear many concerns from our patients receiving orthodontic treatment. It's not uncommon to hear things like *"How long do you have to wear my braces?"*, *"Will they hurt?"*, *"Will my wisdom teeth affect anything?"*

Wait, did you say wisdom teeth?

I did! Wisdom teeth might not be on your radar, but a lot of our patients are very concerned about how their wisdom teeth can affect the outcome of their newly straighten smile. Some patients start to worry when they see their wisdom teeth beginning to emerge, thinking that they will mess up all the treatment they just underwent or are still finishing up.

Is this something to worry about? Can teeth exert enough pressure to move the teeth that are around them? Your worries are justifiable, but we've got you covered! Let's look at how wisdom teeth can affect orthodontic treatment!

First of all, what are wisdom teeth?

Wisdom teeth are the third set of adult molars. They usually make an appearance between the ages of 17–21. Some have theirs come in completely, while others' only come in partially. There are even a few people whose wisdom teeth don't come in at all!

Are wisdom teeth going to affect your smile?

Around the time that wisdom teeth start to come in, many patients will notice a "relapse" in their teeth positions. Are wisdom teeth really the reason for this shift?

You might find this surprising, but studies show that wisdom teeth are not to blame! Most people assume that because wisdom teeth grow in sideways that they must exert quite a bit of pressure on the teeth next to them and cause teeth to shift. However, research has shown that wisdom teeth do not exert the amount of pressure needed to move the teeth in front of them to cause the shift. Researchers place sensors between patients' teeth and observed the pressure on them, both with and without wisdom teeth present. There was no visible difference. So, if wisdom teeth don't cause your teeth to shift in your late teens and early twenties, then what does?

The answer no one wants to hear: We get older!

It's perfectly normal for our teeth to start to change as we get older. They might begin to overlap as part of a natural drifting that occurs, moving teeth forward slightly. As they begin to overlap, the upper teeth will sometimes press the lower teeth inward toward the tongue. Also, around this time of life, the jaw does undergo a growth spurt which can also move teeth into some less than desirable positions.

So, if you've ever wondered why we encourage you to wear your retainer so much, now you know! Wearing your retainer is the best defense to help your teeth stay as straight as they were when you finished your orthodontic treatment!

A Little Wisdom about Wisdom Teeth

Even though wisdom teeth might not affect your newly straighten smile, there are a few oral health concerns you might want to keep in mind if yours are growing in. These concerns can cause some oral health issues:

- If wisdom teeth only emerge partially, a flap of skin can potential form that partially covers the tooth and has a bad habit of trapping food. This can cause gum infection and tooth decay if it is not taken care of.

- Some people don't have enough room in their mouth for their wisdom teeth to fully emerge. When this happens, they often end up impacted. This means that they can break through the surface and get stuck in your jaws and gums, which can cause some discomfort.

- If the they do become impacted, painful cysts can sometimes form on the gums. These cysts can sometimes cause infection and decay to the tooth roots surrounding them.

- Wisdom teeth often emerge sideways or at an awkward angle. If this happens they can rub against the inside of the cheeks and cause discomfort.

One of the biggest concerns we see with wisdom teeth is that many patients don't have enough room for them to come in comfortably. Even if there is enough room for their wisdom teeth, the back of the mouth is usually so crowded that brushing and flossing them proves to be very difficult. This is one of the leading causes of tooth decay and gum infection in the back of the mouth.

Don't skip the retainer!

If you have already had orthodontic treatment, the best thing that you can do to keep your teeth from shifting is wearing your retainer consistently. If you notice your wisdom teeth starting to emerge, give us a call to avoid any of the potential problems that come with impacted or partially emerged wisdom teeth. You should also continue to schedule regular appointments with us or your dentist even after your orthodontic treatment is finished.

To wrap it all up...

Thankfully, problems with overcrowding can be diagnosed long before wisdom teeth ever make their appearance. Once they get close enough to the surface, they can be easily extracted to prevent further complications.

If you're worried about your wisdom teeth coming in during your orthodontic treatment, don't be! Wisdom teeth can't easily be removed while also having braces, so you don't have to worry about how they will affect your treatment. Your treatment will continue uninterrupted!

Not every person has to have their wisdom teeth removed. If you're one of the lucky ones not experiencing problems with yours, then there is no need to have them extracted.

Once again, we cannot emphasize enough how important it is to continuously wear your retainer after finishing up your orthodontic treatment. It's the only sure-fire way to keep your teeth looking as straight as they did when you finished your treatment. If you start to notice that yours is feeling tighter than normal or that there's a bit of pressure in the back of your mouth, schedule a visit with us so that we can determine whether or not it is your wisdom teeth coming in.

CHAPTER 13

Now That You Have Reached Your Smile... Let's Celebrate!

Having to wear braces can last for six months to two years or more in certain cases. During the time your child has them, they may have moved from child to preteen or preteen to teen, at times felt embarrassed by having them, and possibly missed out on some things. They probably gave up favorite foods and snacks. They at least had to be super-conscious of what they ate and didn't eat. It's been a long time since they could sink their teeth into an apple!

You endured whatever complaining there was. You traded time to the office visits. You dealt with the "uh-oh!" and "now what did you do?" emergencies if there were any. And, of course, you paid the bill.

We like to see our patients celebrate getting their braces off. There are so many ways your child can celebrate, everything from writing a journal about their experience to recording a video that shares their experience and shows their new look.

Here are a few options your child may want to consider:

- **Throw a party.** Throwing a "braces are off" party is a great way to celebrate. They can invite their friends over, put out the foods that they've been longing for, and they can enjoy showing off those new straight teeth. His friends will love being able to take part in the celebration.

- **Plan a photo shoot.** Your child deserves to show the world his new beautiful smile! Plan a photo shoot, so he can be one-on-one with a photographer and put his best smile forward. He'll get some great shots and can show all his friends on social media his new look.

- **Chew some gum.** Your child might have wanted to have gum for the longest time. Although it's not the best habit, she can take an afternoon to chew some gum and feel guilt and worry free. Chew to your heart's content!

- **Go caramel.** Now is the time your child can sink his teeth into something like a caramel apple. No more avoiding the caramel and cutting the apple into bite-sized pieces. Nope, he can actually eat a full caramel apple, right off the stick! He can get one at the mall or a carnival or even make them himself. Either way, he'll love being able to bite into that sticky, gooey sweetness worry free!

- **Picnic in the park.** Weather permitting, a picnic in the park will make for a fun celebration. Take some of your child's favorite outdoor games, invite the friends, and have a cooler filled with icy drinks. On the grill, you can plan for things like corn on the cob that your child had to largely avoid while having her braces. It will make for a memorable afternoon.

- **Have a potluck dinner.** Have your child's friends and family each bring a dish people with braces have to take precaution with. This will give them the chance to learn a little more about what you went through, and it'll be fun to see what options they come up with. Ask each of the guests to write down a comment about your child with or without her braces. Your potluck will be filled with interesting dishes, laughs, and a good time.

- **Relax.** What could be better than spending a couple of hours being pampered, or perhaps a round of golf or fishing out on the lake? Not much! Take your child out—celebrate them making it through their treatment. They'll walk out feeling and looking great.

Doing some of these things, such as chewing gum, may still not be good for your child's teeth or their body overall. But doing it on a special occasion, and not making a habit out of it, won't cause any harm.

CHAPTER 14

What About *My* Smile?

Mom, Dad, I'm *not* going to kid you: if braces and/or orthodontic treatment was advised when you were eight or ten or twelve and, for whatever reason, it didn't happen, and you now have misaligned teeth, periodontal problems because of them, a smile you often hide, or jaw/TMJ pain, it may not be an easy fix. It may *not* even be fixable with orthodontics or braces. But often, to the surprise of adults, braces including invisible braces can do a significant amount of good for people thirty, forty, or even fifty years old. You may still be able to go from an embarrassing smile you often hide to a beautiful smile you love. You'll also be able to enjoy better oral health, gently and gradually over six to twelve months without having teeth pulled and without surgery. Many adults see ten years of age disappear from their faces.

The only way to know what the options are is with a complete, expert orthodontic exam.

At my office, we do not actively seek adult patients, but we treat a lot of parents of patients, just like you, and a number of them come from referrals. You can arrange for your exam by speaking to any of the treatment coordinators at the office.

> **After years of being told I needed surgery, my results are amazing without it. I'm finally able to smile in holiday photos.** — Michael R.

It's important to get your son or daughter the orthodontic care they need at the earliest time they are known to need it and for it to be the best care available. When that doesn't happen, it often comes around to really bite that person later in life!

Please don't ask them to hide their smile!

Call us at 573-212-8723 or go to www.bowenortho.com to schedule your own Customized Smile Analysis.

FAQS

Here is a handy resource guide of frequently asked questions and orthodontic terminology, many of which are answered throughout the book.

What might happen if your child's mouth doesn't quite "fit"?
The fact is, the sooner you straighten your child's smile, the faster it will develop as it should: straight, clean, and healthy!

Who are some famous faces who've worn braces?
Gwen Stefani. Prince Harry. Drew Barrymore. Tom Cruise. Dakota Fanning. Danny Glover.

Can I see what my child's straight teeth might look like before the procedure is done?
Yes! Digital pictures are often used to portray what the child's teeth might look like once the braces have been removed.

Will I be able to afford my child's braces?
Not only are most orthodontic procedures cheaper than ever, but insurance, payment plans, and a variety of other financing options make braces more affordable than they've ever been.

Will getting braces be painful for my child?
Not anymore! Modern technology—and choosing the right orthodontist—can ensure that your child enjoys a pain-free orthodontic experience.

How much school will my child miss because of braces?
Not much, actually. After initial visits and, barring the actual procedure itself, most visits and/or adjustments are routine and can take anywhere from 15 to 45 minutes.

Is it really such a big deal if my child has crooked teeth?
Unfortunately, yes. Eroding, crooked, or unaligned smiles can take time to happen, but the time to act is now. Orthodontic irregularities don't just heal on their own or "go away" if you ignore them.

What are some of the warning signs that my child might need to go to the orthodontist?

There are many, but here are a few of the most common: early or late loss of teeth, protruding teeth, grinding or clenching of teeth, and speech difficulty.

What kind of "side effects" are caused by crooked teeth?

Some of the more frequent ones I see include headaches, toothaches, mouth breathing, chipped or worn down teeth, snoring, and drooling.

What makes an orthodontist more qualified than a dentist?

Orthodontists are dental specialists who have completed two to three years of additional education beyond dental school to learn the proper way to align teeth and jaws.

Why should I choose a specialist for my child's orthodontic care?

Unique treatment requirements and otherwise difficult bite problems are common, everyday scenarios for your orthodontist. In the interest of receiving the most efficient and effective orthodontic treatment possible, choose an orthodontic specialist.

How do I know if my doctor is an orthodontist?

Only orthodontists can belong to the American Association of Orthodontists (AAO).

What is a treatment coordinator?

During your initial consultation(s), you will usually be assigned a patient contact person—we call this person a "treatment coordinator" in our office—with whom to schedule appointments, confer with rescheduling and, of course, answer any and all questions you may have.

Why are follow-up visits important?

These are wonderful opportunities to either a.) ask questions you may have missed the first time or b.) get further details from your orthodontist him- or herself.

Why is early treatment so important?

Age seven is the earliest time your orthodontist can determine future jaw and tooth alignment. That's because, at the age of seven, your child's upper and lower permanent front teeth are developing. These teeth set the stage for future jaw position and serious problems can develop if they come into the wrong position.

Is there such a thing as a child being too old for braces?

Actually, there is. Case in point: waiting to take your child to the orthodontist until they are twelve or thirteen can be very risky.

What if I don't believe in early orthodontics?

Well, you're entitled to your opinion, but this is like saying you don't believe in the sun. You can hide from it, pretend it's not there, or refuse to acknowledge it, but the simple fact remains. If you're not aware of the potential risks, you can get burnt.

Will my child actually need braces at seven?

Probably not. While I inform parents their child needs an initial exam at age seven, I also mention that most children will not need braces until eleven to thirteen years of age.

What is a crossbite?

When the upper and lower teeth grow at different rates, or even when the lower jaw grows disproportionately with the upper jaw, something known as a "crossbite" can occur.

Where should I start to look for treatment if I'm concerned about my child's jaw development?

If you suspect your child might have a crossbite or other issues, approach your family dentist and ask about orthodontics.

Why should I address a crossbite?

Crossbites can lead to pain, discomfort, and lack of confidence as your child begins to feel insecure or even ostracized because of this very treatable, very normal series of jaw and teeth developments.

What is Invisalign?

The Invisalign system is the virtually invisible way to straighten your teeth and achieve the dazzling smile you've always dreamed of. Using advanced 3-D computer-imaging technology, Invisalign depicts your complete treatment plan, from the initial position of your teeth to the final desired position.

What are the primary benefits of Invisalign?

Like the word that inspired them, Invisalign aligners are practically clear; or as close to "invisible" as one can get. No one may even notice you're wearing these virtually invisible braces, making Invisalign a seamless fit with your lifestyle and day-to-day interactions with others.

How do I get started with Invisalign?

It's simple: just make an appointment with your local orthodontist for an initial consultation. Most doctors will offer a free initial consultation to see if you are a good candidate for Invisalign.

How will Invisalign effectively move my teeth?

Aligners are the foundation for, and work in unison with, the Invisalign system. Like brackets and arch wires are to braces, Invisalign aligners move teeth by using the appropriate placement of controlled force on your child's teeth.

How many patients are being treated with Invisalign?

More than one million patients worldwide have been treated with Invisalign. The number of Invisalign smiles grows daily.

Is Invisalign appropriate for my child?

Yes, especially because Invisalign now has a system designed specifically for teens!

How does Invisalign Teen work?

Aligners snap on your teeth easily. They are comfortable and practically invisible. Invisalign Teen allows permanent teeth to grow and gently and continuously moves your teeth in small increments. Aligners are worn for about two weeks, then you swap them for a new pair.

Why are metal braces still so popular?

Metal braces are very strong and can withstand most types of treatment. Today's metal braces are smaller, sleeker, and more polished than ever before.

Are so-called "clear braces" effective?

Ceramic braces are very strong and generally do not stain. Two popular brands are Clarity, made by 3M Unitek, and Empower made by American Orthodontics. Adults like to choose ceramic braces because they "blend in" with the teeth and are less noticeable than metal. These are the types of braces actor Tom Cruise had.

Are clear braces appropriate for adults?

Absolutely! Adults of all ages can enjoy the same cosmetic and health benefits of properly aligned teeth with Empower system and Clarity braces.

What are some of my payment options in addition to insurance?

One way many patients pay for their procedures is by utilizing the benefits of what is known as "flex spending," where their employer matches their spending commitment.

What if my child has a "braces emergency" before or after office hours?

If you are experiencing an orthodontic emergency that can't wait for regular office hours, most orthodontic offices have a special number to call, either before, during, or after business hours. If this information isn't given to you readily, ask how your doctor's office handles emergencies.

Can a salt water rinse help deal with irritation caused by braces?

Absolutely; warm saltwater rinses soothe the cheek lining, which can get aggravated by your child's braces.

How do I make a salt water rinse?

To make a salt water rinse, mix ½ teaspoon of table salt in one cup of warm water. Stir until the salt is completely dissolved. Gently swish about ¼ of the cup in your mouth for 30 seconds. Make sure you force the water over the areas that feel sore. Then spit the water into the sink. Repeat until the entire cup is gone.

What if my child plays sports and needs a mouth guard?

The best advice for patients or parents looking for a mouth guard can be obtained from your pediatrician, dentist, pediatric dentist, orthodontist or oral surgeon. All of these specialists are uniquely trained to offer customized advice in order to help you prevent a sports-related dental or facial injury.

What about brushing with braces?

Here are some simple tips you can share with your child for the best results when brushing with braces on:

- Brush your teeth with a medium nylon toothbrush after you eat and before bed.

- Brush, rinse, and look; if you find any areas that are not clean, brush them again.

- Brush your gums as you brush your teeth (massage and stimulate).

- If no toothpaste is available, brush without.

- If you are unable to brush, rinse your mouth vigorously with water.

- Replace your old toothbrush when it gets worn out.

- It is absolutely essential that you continue regular visits to your family dentist for checkups and cleanings throughout your orthodontic treatment!

What type of foods should my child avoid while wearing braces?

There are four main types of food your child should avoid while wearing braces: **hard foods**, like ice, popcorn, peanut brittle, rock candy, and corn on the cob; **sticky foods,** like caramels, bubble gum, taffy, and suckers; **chewy foods,** like pizza crust, crusty breads, beef jerky, and gummy bears; and **sugary foods and drinks,** like cake, ice cream, cookies, pie, candy, and soda pop.

Why are retainers so important?

As we age, teeth naturally shift to the middle and crowd. Combined with late growth of the lower jaw, shifting of the teeth is expected following orthodontic treatment. Therefore, retainers are extremely important in the maintenance of your new smile following orthodontic treatment.

THE NEXT STEP:
Your Customized Smile Analysis

When you are ready, I urge you to schedule your **Customized Smile Analysis**, with a complimentary consultation; safe, digital x-rays (a $249 value) and exam; and report to you and your son or daughter—*all without cost or obligation.*

Call us at 573-212-8723 or go to www.bowenortho.com to schedule your own Customized Smile Analysis.

RESOURCES

Before or after your consultation, you may want more information for yourself or your son or daughter. The following websites provide valuable insight to help you make the right decision for your child.

Braces.org is the "all about braces site" of the American Association of Orthodontists. This is the official regulatory body and professional association of orthodontists, and only orthodontists (not dentists) can be members. Here you will receive accurate, up-to-date information on orthodontics.

ExcellenceInOrthodontics.org is the elite association of orthodontists subscribing to a pledge of clinical and customer services excellence. A complete collection of information for patients and parents can be found here.

ABOUT THE AUTHOR

Dr. Thomas B Bowen is a speaker, teacher, author and orthodontic specialist. Dr. Bowen graduated Magna Cum Laude from the University of Central Florida and then received his doctorate in dentistry from the University of Alabama School of Dentistry. He was a recipient of the Army's Health Scholarship Program. After serving 4 years as a captain in the US Army both in the United States and overseas, he spent 10 years in private practice in Asheville, NC. After going back to residency and earning his Masters degree in orthodontics and dentofacial orthopedics, he founded Bowen Orthodontics in Rolla and St. Robert, MO. Dr. Bowen also has four children of his own, 3 sons and a daughter. Dr. Bowen's vision is to change lives, advance the profession of orthodontics and support his community.

The core focus of Dr. Bowen and his team is to help children and adults "Reach Their Smile." More than that he believes orthodontics is more than just creating smiles. It is about forming strong relationships and friendships with patients, families, dental colleagues, and the community. He also serves as the president of the Ozark Dental Society and maintains memberships with both professional organizations and community groups.

Dr. Bowen supports the local community by giving grants to both teachers and students and provides free orthodontic care through the program Smiles Change Lives.

www.ingramcontent.com/pod-product-compliance
Lightning Source LLC
Chambersburg PA
CBHW070813280326
41934CB00012B/3179